I0439790

Lent And Fasting
The Foundation of Good Health
Recipe Book

The Cleansing Of Body And Soul

Demetra S. Gerontakis

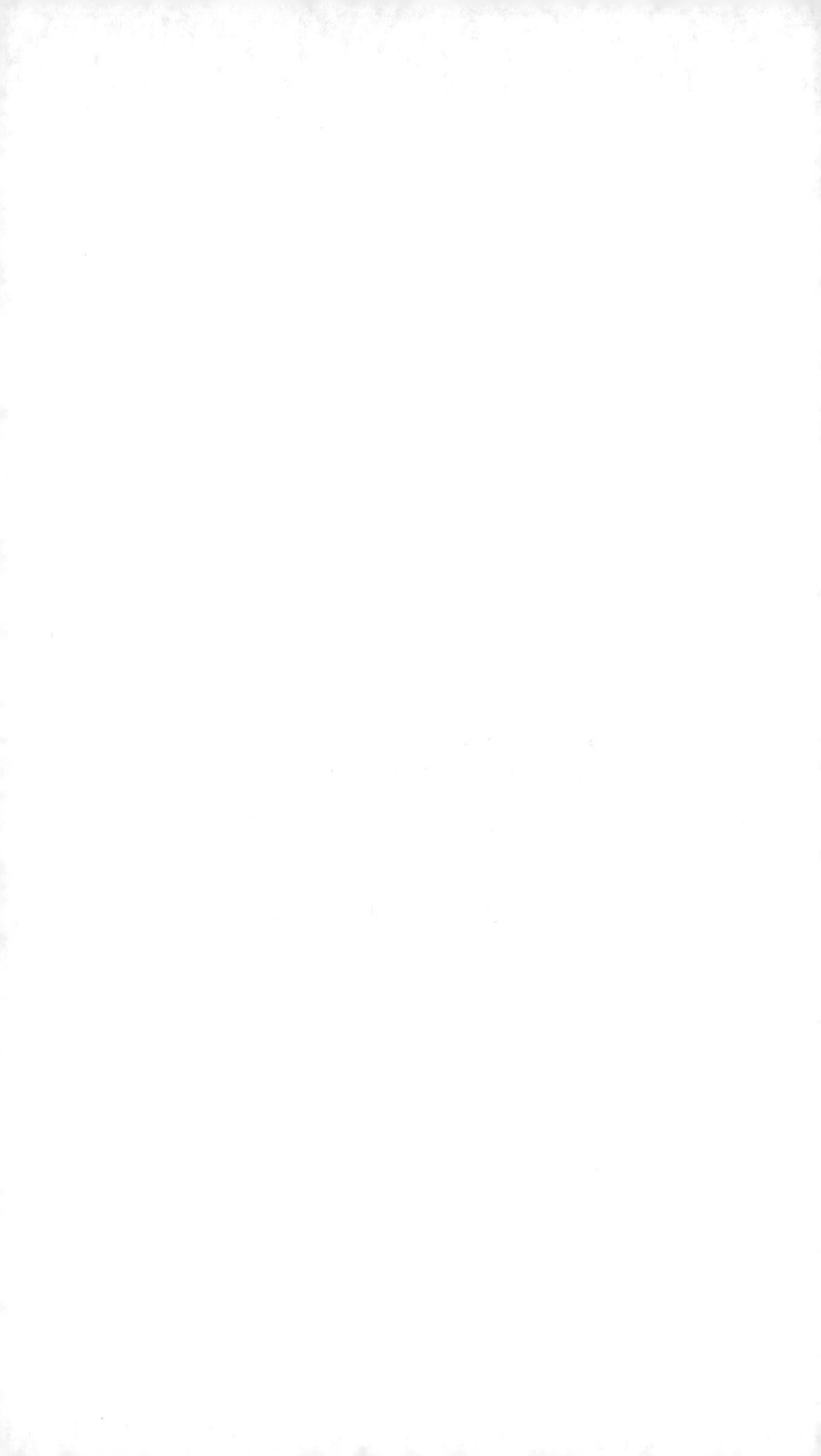

CONTENTS

Pasta Dishes

Mushroom Macaroni
Eggplant and Pasta
Vegetable pasta soufflé

Legume Dishes
Dried kidney beans with rice casserole
Black-eyed beans and octopus

Nutritious snack mix

INTRODUCTION

Did you know that fasting can help fight against Brain disease such as Alzheimer's and Parkinson's? That fasting helps the immune system work more efficiently, allowing more oxygen and white blood cells to flow through the body, helping it to burn more fat and increase energy which allows other healing functions? Some even claim that a cancer patient can actually "starve" a tumor therefore killing the cell. Fasting decreases insulin levels, burns fat, promotes weight loss. Even philosophers have emphasized on the subject of fasting. A word of warning: whether someone goes on a diet or would like to fast for some time span short or long it is strongly advised that you ask your doctor before starting either as it maybe dangerous to diet or fast, when there are health issues.

Ancient Greek Philosophy and Fasting.

"Everyone has a physician inside him or her; we just have to help it in its work. The natural healing force within each one of us is the greatest force in getting well. Our food should be our medicine. Our medicine should be our food. But to eat when you are sick is to feed your sickness."

Hippocrates

"Instead of using medicine, rather, fast a day."

Plutarch

Pythagoras (580-500 years. BC), Greek philosopher and mathematician, founder of the famous school of philosophy, systematically starved for 40 days, rightly believing that it increases the mental perception and creativity. He demanded strict 40-day fast on water alone from each of his numerous disciples and followers

Plato (427-347 years BC), disciple of Socrates, divided medicine into "true", which really gives health, and "false", which gives only the "phantom of health." The first one included treatments by fasting and diet, air and sun.

The Holy fathers Of Christianity have taught through out the ages about the benefits that fasting has on both body and soul.

***

Fasting of the body is food for the soul.

***

Fasting is wonderful, because it tramples our sins like a dirty weed, while it cultivates and raises truth like a flower.

***

The reason that fasting has an effect on the spirits of evil rests in its powerful effect on our own spirit. A body subdued by fasting brings the human spirit freedom, strength, sobriety, purity, and keen discernment.

***

Seest thou what fasting does: it heals illnesses, drives out demons, removes wicked thoughts, makes the heart pure. If someone has even been seized by an impure spirit, let him know that this kind, according to the word of the Lord, *"goeth not out but by prayer and fasting"* (Matthew 17:21).

***

True fasting lies is rejecting evil, holding one's tongue, suppressing one's hatred, and banishing one's lust, evil words, lying, and betrayal of vows.

***

'In proportion as the body grows fat, so does the soul wither away.'

***

References: Holy Hierarch John Chrysostom, Holy Righteous John of Kronstadt, Saint Athanasius the Great, Holy Hierarch Basil the Great Abba Daniel of Sketis:

THE ORIGIN OF FASTING

The First and oldest command given to us by God is the command of fasting.

The LORD God commanded the man, saying, "From any tree of the garden you may eat freely; but from the tree of the knowledge of good and evil you shall not eat, for in the day that you eat from it you will surely die." (Genesis 2:17)

Though out the bible fasting is mentioned over and over again. Even Jesus fasted for forty days.

Then Jesus was led up by the Spirit into the wilderness to be tempted by the devil. And after He had fasted forty days and forty nights, He then became hungry.(Matthew 4:2)

The meaning of Lent

Fasting has been practiced by pagan religions, Judaism and Christianity. It is one of the most important factors of religious life. In some religions, fasting means complete abstention from all food for a period of time. In others, it means not eating certain foods such as meat, fish poultry and dairy products for a few days to over a month. But what is Lent exactly? Lent: in the Christian religion is an annual season of fasting and penitence. Fasting: promotes the cleansing of the body and the clearing of the fogginess of the mind. As a result, both body and mind stay alert. Finally, Fasting joins the body and mind into a deeper relationship with the soul cleansing it too, and awakening it from its lethargy.

Fasting from certain foods benefits our Health

Fasting is an ancient tradition practiced from the beginning of time for curing illnesses, to rejuvenate, cleanse and strengthen the body but also to gain clarity. It helps the body to detoxify by attacking all kinds of harmful toxins. Keeping away from all meat products, fish, poultry and all dairy products is beneficial to the body's whole mechanism.

In opposite, eating raw fruit, vegetables, seeds and nuts as well as vegetable broths, lightly steamed vegetables and fresh fruit juices which are essential for the body to detoxify can have positive effects such as lowering cholesterol and high blood pressure.

Adding legumes such as lentil, peas, navy, red, black or even lima beans help in detoxification but also to keep up energy levels.

Let's not forget whole grains used in our bread and cake recipes as well as sesame, walnuts. Almonds, raisins, dried fruit and shelled peanuts.

Learning to abstain from meat and dairy groups and indulge in the grain, fruit and vegetable group can benefit our body's health greatly.

Lastly, we must keep in mind that fasting also means to minimize quantities.

Recipes

Pumpkin or squash pie

Ingredients: 2.20 lbs of shredded pumpkin or squash drained of all juices.
1 cup black raisins
1 cup extra virgin olive oil
1 cup sugar
2/3 cups corn meal
2 tsps dried ground mint leaves
½ tsp salt
1 package filo dough (8 sheets)
Extra oil for basting

Mix all ingredients thoroughly in a large bowl. Oil a baking pan and layer filo dough sheets one by one basting each one with sunflower or corn oil. Once you have layered 4 sheets of filo dough spread your mix evenly into the dough. Continue to layer the remaining four sheets of filo dough in the same manner. Cut into pieces before baking so that the dough doesn't crust won't crumble after cooking. Spray with water once or twice during the baking process. Bake at medium heat for 45 min. Optional: can be done with homemade dough.

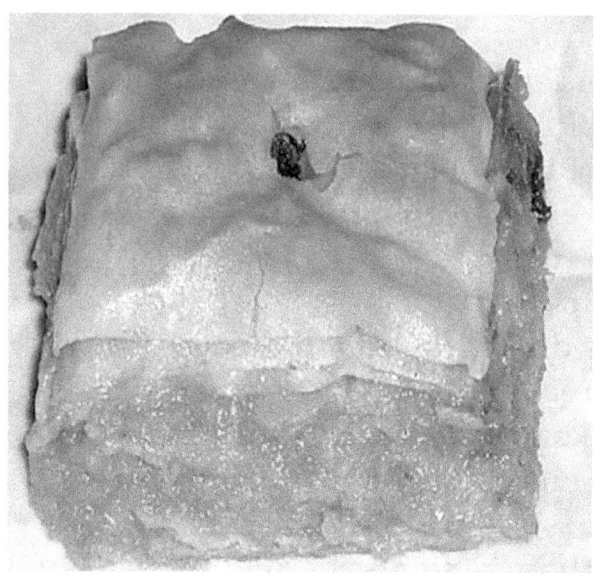

Cabbage pie

Ingedients: 1 3 lb white cabbage
2 large carrots 1 cup parsley
1 slice garlic ½ cup short grin white rice
Juice from half a lemon
Salt to taste, 1 tsp sweet pepper powder
(paprika) 1 cup extra virgin olive oil
1 package filo dough.In a bowl mix
finely chopped parsley,garlic,shredded
cabbage and shredded carrots with
lemon juice oil an spices. After mixing
well add rice and mix until it is spread
evenly. . Oil a baking pan and layer filo
dough sheets one by one basting each
one with sunflower or corn oil. Once
you have layered 4 sheets of filo dough
spread your mix evenly into the dough.
Continue to layer the remaining four
sheets of filo dough in the same manner.
Cut into pieces before baking so that the
dough doesn't crust won't crumble after
cooking. Spray with water once or twice
during the baking process. Bake at
medium heat for 75 min. Optional: can
be done with homemade dough.

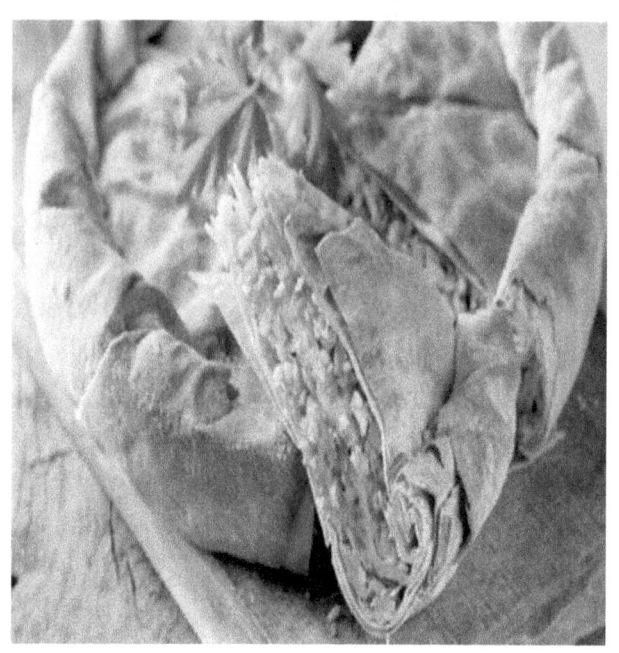

Spinach and Leek Pie

Ingredients:

1 ½ lb fresh spinach
2 leeks
8-10 chard leaves
1 bunch of fresh baby onions
1 bunch of fresh dill
1 cup extra virgin olive oil
2/3 cup cornmeal
4-5 fresh mint leaves (optional)
Salt and pepper to taste
Wash all vegetables thoroughly. Put aside until drained. Chop all vegetables as thin as possible and put into a large bowl. Add oil, cornmeal salt and pepper and mix. Oil a baking pan and layer filo dough sheets one by one basting each one with sunflower or corn oil.

Once you have layered 4 sheets of filo dough spread your mix evenly into the dough. Continue to layer the remaining four sheets of filo dough in the same manner. Cut into pieces before baking so that the dough doesn't crust won't crumble after cooking. Spray with water once or twice during the baking process. Bake at medium heat for 75 min. Optional: can be done with homemade dough.

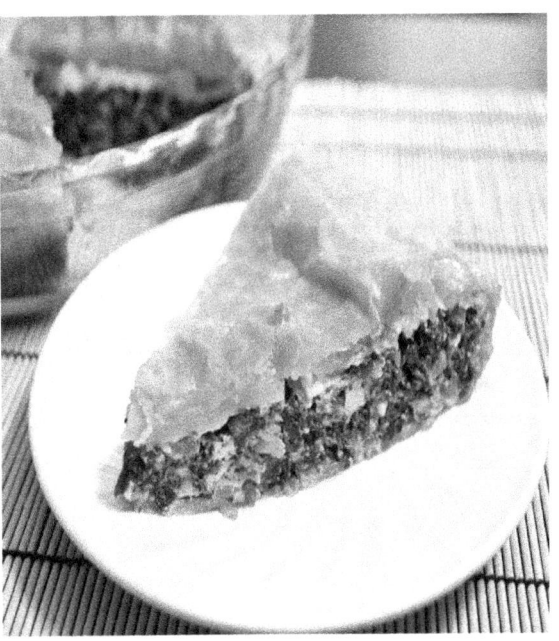

Chickpea Patties

Ingredients: 1 lb of chickpeas
1 small bunch of parsley
3 garlic cloves, 1 bunch of baby green onions, salt and spices of choice.
Frying oil.
Preparation: On the previous night, soak the chickpeas in a bowl with tap water and a teaspoon of salt. They must be covered in water two times over. Next day strain and put them into the blender to make them mashed. Add all other finely chopped veggies and spices and then form small flat patties. Let the patties sit in the refrigerator for half hour. Put oil in a frying pan over <u>low</u> heat and fry patties slowly as to make sure they cook evenly well on both sides.

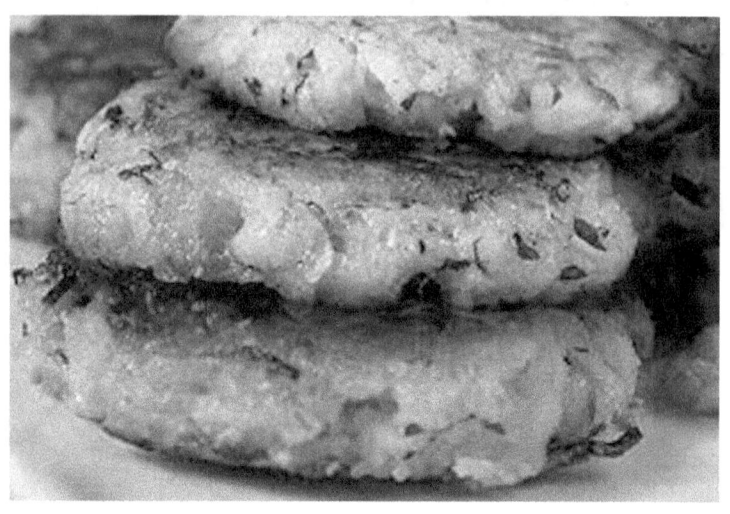

Potato patties

Ingredients: 2 ½ lbs potatoes
1 cup finely chopped parsley
1 large white onion finely chopped
½ lb grated soy cheese
Salt and pepper to taste
3 tablespoons extra virgin olive oil
Frying oil
Flour

Boil potatoes and mash. Add all other ingredients except for flour; you will need that to fry. Shape your potato dough into patties and let them sit in refrigerator for ½ hr. Heat oil in frying pan at medium. Flour and shake off access flour and then place into frying pan. Fry evenly on both sides.

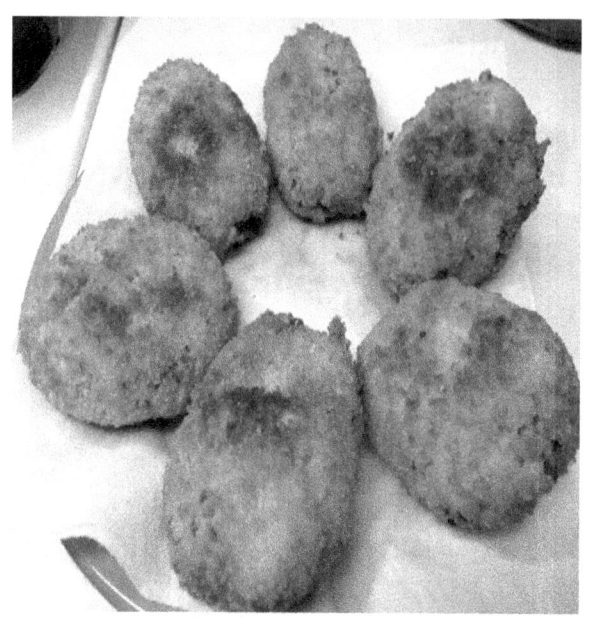

Mushroom Patties

Ingredients: 1 lb mushrooms
1 medium red onion
5 tablespoons of farina flour
2 medium boiled potatoes
Salt, pepper
½ cup fresh dill finely chopped
Frying oil

Finely chop mushrooms. Mash potatoes, add all ingredients and form small patties about 3 or 4 centimeters wide.

Heat oil in frying pan over medium heat. Fry both sides evenly.

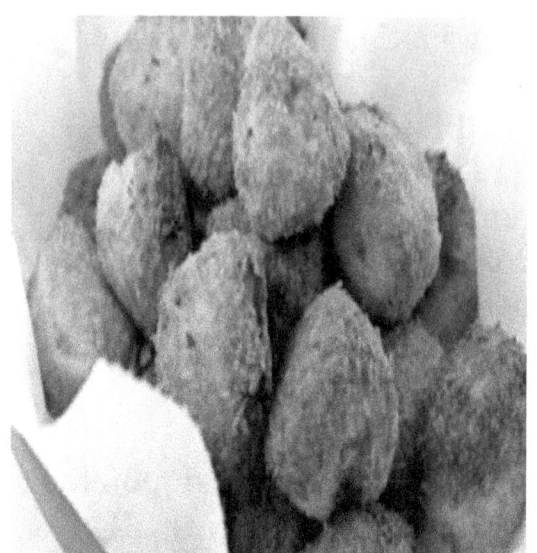

Cabbage in Tomato Sauce

Ingredients: 1 Small head of cabbage approximately 18-20 centimeters wide.
1 cup extra virgin olive oil
2 small leeks
1 medium red onion
1 cup of fresh tomato sauce or store bought if preferred
3 medium tomatoes skinned and chopped finely
½ cup red wine
Salt
½ tsp sweet chili pepper, some water.
Wash cabbage and cut into large pieces. In a large saucepan boil some water and place cabbage to boil for 10 minutes. Strain. In another saucepan; sauté onion and leeks until withered and then add chopped tomato and sauce. Simmer for 5 minutes. Add all other ingredients including cabbage. Add 2 cups water and simmer at medium heat until most juices have drained and a nice sauce is left.

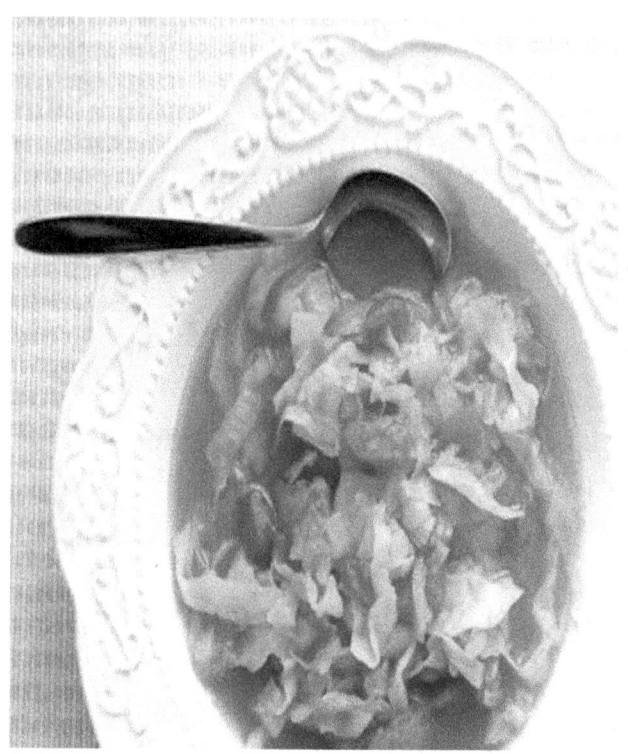

Stuffed Peppers with Mushrooms

Ingredients: 6 large sweet peppers
2 ½ cups of chopped mushrooms
2 fresh ripe grated tomatoes
1 large grated onion
1/2 cup parsley
1clove of garlic finely chopped
Salt and pepper
½ tsp sugar
1 cup olive oil
2 tblsp of short grain white rice for each pepper. (12 tblsp)
In sauce pan sauté in oil in order; onion, parsley, garlic, mushrooms and last tomatoes and seasonings. Once withered add rice and pull off heat. Set aside. Wash and dry sweet peppers and slice along one side allowing space enough to stuff. Stuff each one with mix and place neatly into baking pan. Baking pan should be small as to perfectly fit peppers tightly. Add 350 ml water a little salt and bake at medium heat for an hour covered with foil paper. Last 5 minutes uncover pan to gain color.

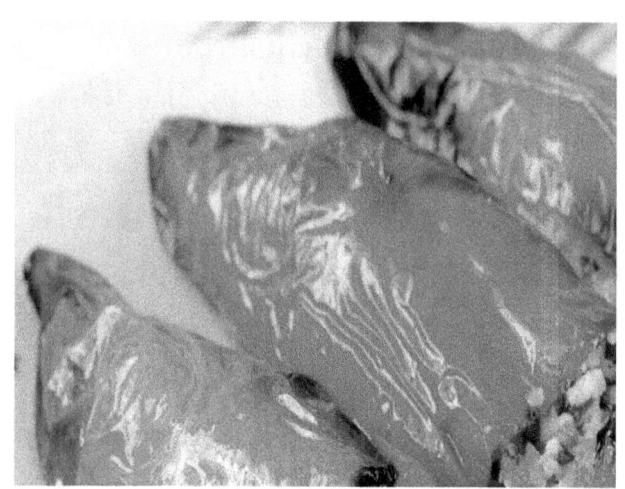

Leek in Tomato Sauce

Ingredients: 3 ½ lbs of Leeks chopped in round slices
1 cup celery finely chopped
1 cup carrot slices
1 cup fresh baby onions chopped finely
1 cup fresh grated tomato or (canned)
Salt, pepper to taste.
¾ cup extra virgin olive oil

In a large sauce pan put olive oil and sauté onion, carrot and tomato for 5 minutes. Add all other ingredients and seasoning then let simmer for 40 minutes with lid over low heat. Add lemon juice before serving (optional)

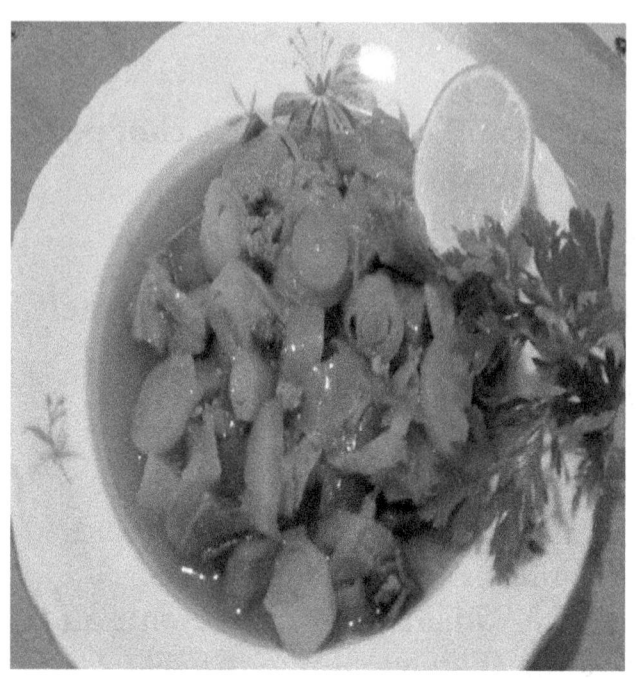

Mushroom Macaroni

1 ½ lb elbow, tube or rice macaroni
1 ½ lb mushrooms chopped slices
1 large red onion grated
1 clove garlic chopped finely
1sweet pepper chopped finely
Two ripe tomatoes grated
Salt
Sweet chili pepper
½ cup extra virgin olive oil

Sauté onion garlic red pepper and mushrooms in oil for 10 minutes. Add tomato and spices simmer for 10 minute low heat. Add 5 cups of water and bring to boil. Add macaroni and cook over medium heat with lid until all juices are drained.

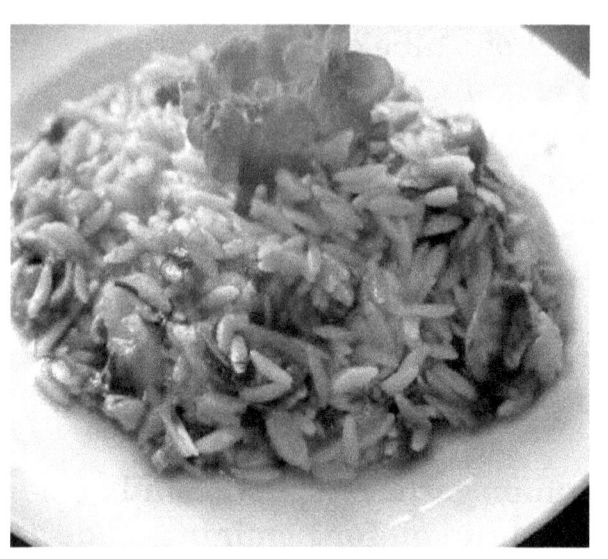

Eggplant and Pasta

Ingredients:

1 lb eggplants
4-5 medium ripe tomatoes
¾ cup extra virgin olive oil
1 clove of garlic
2 carrots
1 onion
1/3 cup red wine
½ tsp sugar
Salt &pepper
1 package of your favorite pasta boiled and strained.

In a medium saucepan add oil, finely chopped carrots, garlic, onion and mince for 5 min. add wine tomatoes and seasonings and simmer 5 more minutes. Add eggplant that has been finely grated or chopped and 1 cup of water. Simmer over low heat with lid until juices are absorbed. Serve over buttered pasta or blend with pasta.

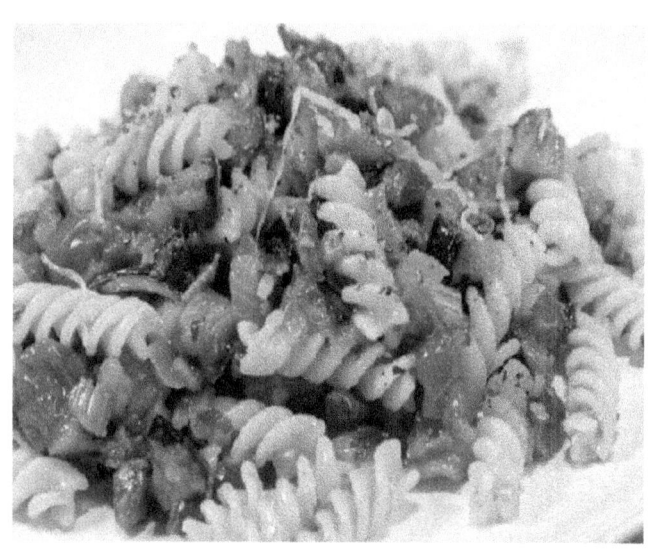

Vegetable Pasta Soufflé

Ingredients: ¼ lb broccoli
½ lb mushrooms
2 carrots
1 garlic clove
1-2 medium zucchini
Salt and pepper
Virgin olive oil ½ cup
1 cup flour
1 stick of margarine (150 gr.)
500 gr. Penne

Chop up all vegetables finely. Sauté lightly in olive oil and seasonings for 20 minutes at low heat. Boil penne al dente and strain. In a large bowl mix penne and vegetables thoroughly. In a medium saucepan melt salted margarine and slowly pour in flour mixing quickly with a mixer while pouring in water until a smooth cream is formed called béchamel.

Pour all vegetables in baking pan along with 1 cup of this cream so that pasta, vegetables and béchamel become one. Spread out the mix evenly in pan and then cover with the rest of the béchamel cream. Bake at medium heat for 45 min. or until nicely brown. Note: let cool for 20 minutes before cutting and serving.

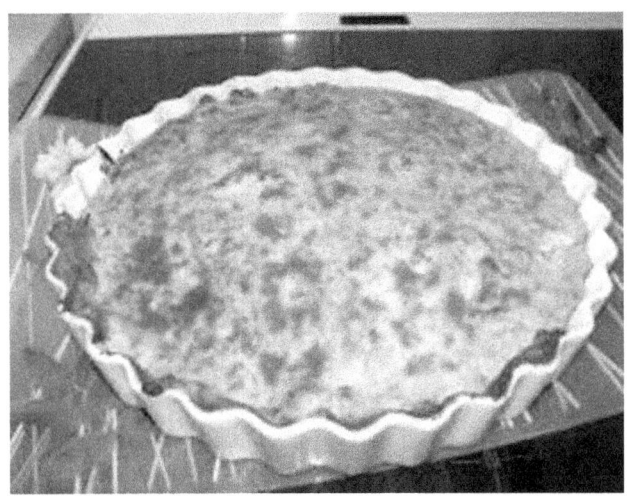

Legumes

Dried kidney beans with rice

Ingredients: 1 lb dried kidney beans soaked for 24 hours prior to cooking.
1 cup olive oil
1 large onion
Salt, red sweet pepper,
One leek
1 cup short grain white rice.

Boil beans in pressure cooker for 1 hr with salt.
When they are almost cooked add rice and cook till rice is done stirring frequently so as not to stick. Sauté finely chopped onion and leek in a skillet until withered. Add red pepper and pour the mix into the beans. Serve hot.

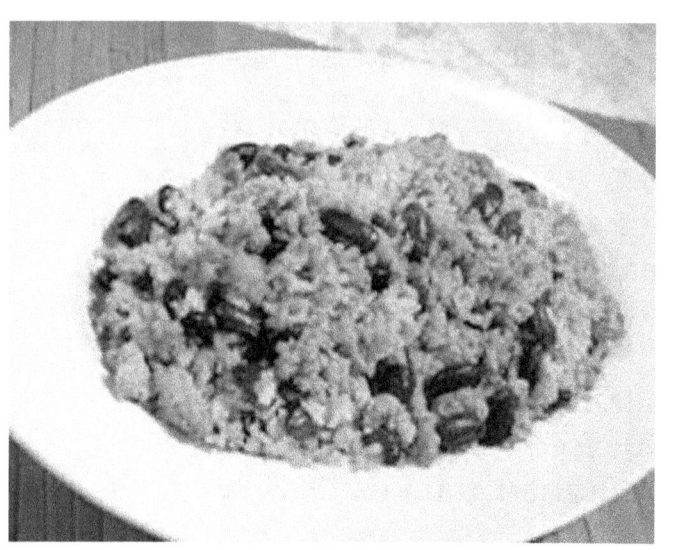

Black-Eyed Beans and Octopus

Ingredients: 2-3 cups boiled black eyed beans strained
1 small octopus about 300 gr. boiled and chopped in small pieces or cubes
4-5 baby green fresh onions finely chopped
1 medium red onion sliced
Salt pepper
1-2 tablespoons red vinegar
½ cup finely chopped parsley
½ cup olive oil
2 dill pickles are optional

In a large bowl mix all ingredients mixing in olive oil and vinegar just before serving.

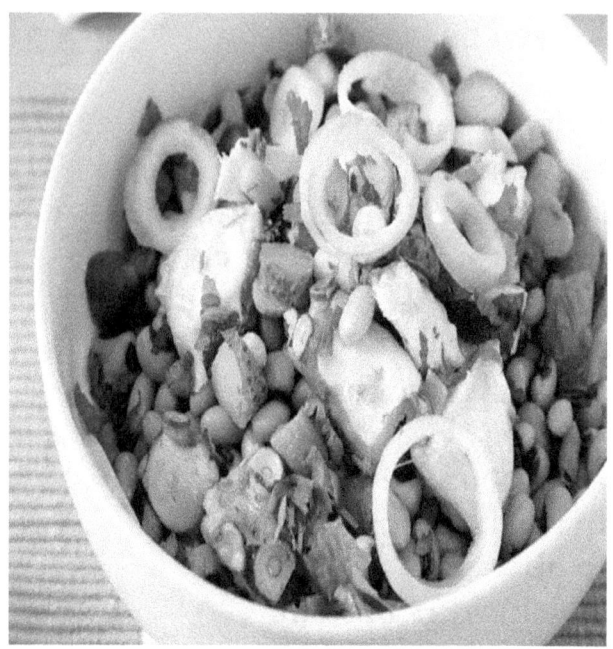

Nutritious snack mix

20 almonds chopped and toasted slightly in a non stick pan
20 walnuts chopped 50 gr sesame seeds toasted
½ cup black raisins
1 cup boiled and drained whole grain wheat kernels
½ tsp cinnamon
3 tblsp sugar
A pinch of salt
½ cup bread crumbs
Pomegranate seeds (optional)

Mix all ingredients serve with a spoon.

Note: Best eaten fresh as grain has the tendency to harden after a day.

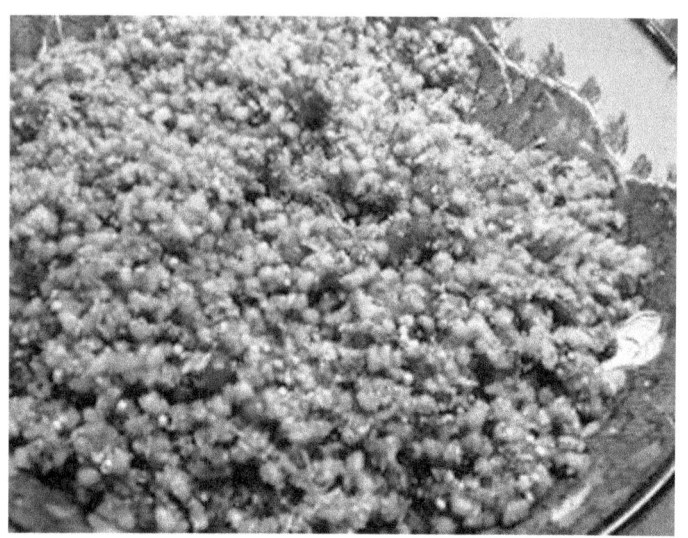

Epilogue

Fasting during Lent can change your life.

***

Fasting just for one week a month can be beneficial to both body and mind.

***

Fasting works miracles for the human body.

***

Health Note: No one should diet or fast without consulting their doctor first

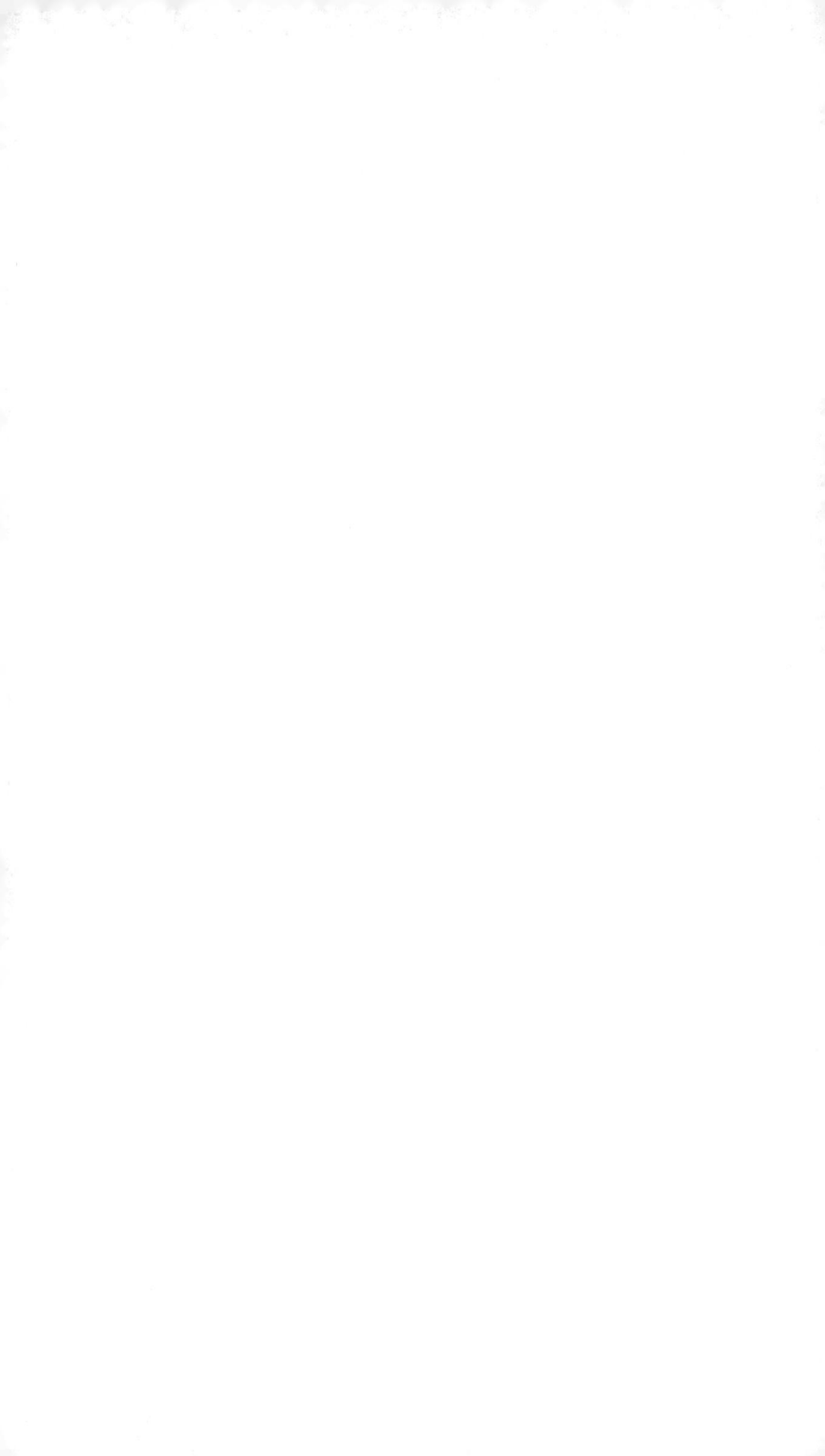